The Hydrogen Sulfide SIBO Guide

Understand the "Third Type" of Bacterial Overgrowth, Rotten-Egg Gas, Flat-Line Breath Tests, and a Practical Low-Sulfur Plan to Calm Your Gut

Cherry B. Johnston

This book is for educational and informational purposes only. It is not medical advice, and it is not a substitute for diagnosis, treatment, or advice from a qualified healthcare professional. Hydrogen sulfide small intestinal bacterial overgrowth, also called intestinal sulfide overproduction, is an area of active clinical research, and the science described here continues to evolve. The author, Cherry B. Johnston, is a registered nurse and researcher, but she is not your clinician and cannot know your history, your medications, or your particular situation. Reading this book does not create a nurse-patient, clinician-patient, or any other professional relationship between the author and the reader. Nothing in these pages should be used to start, stop, or change any medication, supplement, or treatment. Always consult a suitably qualified doctor, dietitian, or specialist before making changes to your diet, your supplements, or your care, and seek prompt medical attention for severe, persistent, or worsening symptoms.

The dietary approaches in this book involve periods of food restriction. Restriction of this kind is not appropriate for everyone. If you have a history of disordered eating, or if reading about food rules provokes anxiety, fear, or a sense of losing control around food, please work through this material with a clinician or a registered dietitian rather than on your own. Reducing the range of foods you eat carries real risks to your nutrition and your relationship with eating, and those risks deserve as much respect as the gut symptoms you are trying to calm.

No outcome is promised or guaranteed, and individual results vary. Any decision about diet, supplements, testing, or treatment remains the responsibility of the reader together with their clinician. Any names, examples, and scenarios in this book are illustrative and composite; they are used only to explain the material and are not intended to describe, represent, harm, or misrepresent any actual person or entity. References to specific tests, products, or organizations are made for the reader's information only and do not constitute an endorsement. The author and publisher have made reasonable efforts to ensure accuracy at the time of writing but assume no responsibility for errors, omissions, or outcomes arising from the use of this material.

First edition, 2026.

ISBN: 979-8-90599-307-7

Table of Contents

Preface

There is a particular kind of quiet that settles over a person when a test comes back normal and they do not feel normal at all.

I have watched it happen many times. Someone sits across from a screen or holds a printout, and the words say no abnormality detected, and instead of relief there is a sinking recognition that the search is not over, only stalled. The bloating is still there. The gas that clears a room is still there. The fatigue that no amount of sleep resolves is still there. And now there is a piece of paper suggesting that perhaps the problem was never real to begin with.

I wrote this book for the people caught in that gap between what the test says and what the body is doing.

My background is in Nursing, not as a gastroenterologist, and I want to be honest about that from the first page. What I bring is not a laboratory or a prescription pad. What I bring is years of sitting with people whose suffering was dismissed because it did not fit a tidy category, and a stubborn belief that being believed is the first thing a person needs before anything else can help. Somewhere along the way, more and more of the people I worked with were carrying gut symptoms alongside everything else, and the same story kept surfacing. The test was negative. The doctor shrugged. The internet offered a hundred contradictory food lists. And underneath it all sat a specific, treatable pattern that almost nobody had named for them.

That pattern is hydrogen sulfide overgrowth, and it is the subject of this book.

I need to be clear about what this book is and is not. It is not a cookbook. The shelf is already crowded with thin recipe collections, some of which, remarkably, include the very foods a person is trying to avoid. It is not a cure, and anyone promising you one should be treated with suspicion. It is not a replacement for a good clinician, and if it does its job well, it will send you toward one better prepared than you were before.

What it is, I hope, is a map. A way of understanding why your breath test may have missed something real, what the sulfur subtype actually looks and feels like once you strip away the myths, how to use a low-sulfur approach as a short and deliberate tool rather than a life sentence, and how to widen your plate again when the time comes. I have tried to write it the way I would explain it to someone sitting across from me who is tired, a little frightened, and out of patience with being told there is nothing wrong.

This isn't just in your head. Let us find out what it is.

Cherry B. Johnston is a Registered Nurse and Researcher

Chapter 1: The Third Gas

Ozias had a folder, and I want to tell you about the folder, because I think you might own one too.

It was a plain plastic folder, the kind you buy in a pack of five, and inside it he kept every test result he had accumulated over three years of trying to find out why his body had turned on him. He brought it to our first conversation and set it on the table between us with the particular care of a man handling evidence, because that is what it was to him. Evidence that he was not making it up. He had a breath test in there, from early on, that had shown hydrogen, and he had been treated for that, and he had gotten better for a while. Then he had gotten worse. A later test came back clean, and he was told his overgrowth had resolved and that whatever remained was just irritable bowel syndrome, something to be lived with rather than solved. He did not believe it, and he was right not to, and the reason he was right is the subject of this entire book.

For most of the modern history of gut overgrowth, the science could count to two. There was hydrogen and there was methane, two gases, two patterns, two boxes into which a suffering gut could be sorted. If your test lit up with one, you had a certain kind of problem. If it lit up with the other, you had a different one. And if it lit up with neither, the working assumption was that you had no overgrowth at all, and the search moved on, or, more often, simply stopped. Ozias had fallen into the gap that opens up when a person has every symptom of a condition and a test that insists they have nothing. What almost nobody had told him was that there was a third gas, one the standard test was never built to see, and that he had very likely been producing it the whole time.

What overgrowth actually is

Let me build this from the ground up, because the whole thing only makes sense against the picture of a gut working properly.

The small intestine is the long, coiled middle stretch of your digestive tract, the part between your stomach and your large intestine, and it is where most of the real work of absorption happens. It is supposed to be a relatively quiet place, at least where bacteria are concerned. Your large intestine teems with a dense and mostly friendly bacterial population, but the small intestine is meant to keep its numbers low, and your body has a set of housekeeping systems that enforce this. Stomach acid sterilizes much of what comes through. Bile and enzymes make the environment inhospitable to squatters. And between meals, a wave of muscular contractions sweeps through, clearing out debris and stray bacteria like a cleaning crew moving through an office after everyone has gone home (Deloose et al., 2012).

Small intestinal bacterial overgrowth, which everyone shortens to SIBO, is what happens when that arrangement breaks down and bacteria pile up in the small intestine in numbers that do not belong there (Pimentel et al., 2020). The bacteria are often not exotic invaders. Frequently they are perfectly ordinary gut organisms that have simply set up shop in the wrong neighborhood. And once they are there, they do what bacteria do. They meet the carbohydrates in your meal before your body has finished absorbing them, and they ferment. Fermentation makes gas. Gas makes bloating, pain, pressure, and bowels that will not behave. This is why a person with SIBO can eat a reasonable meal and inflate within the hour, and why the same meal on a different day lands differently depending on what else is happening down there.

Here is the piece that matters for everything ahead, and it is the piece Ozias had never been told. The gas that fermentation produces is not one single substance. Different microbial communities make different gases, and the gas your particular gut favors turns out to shape both what you feel and whether a standard test can even detect that anything is wrong.

Two gases, and the one they left out

For decades, the breath test measured two gases, and an entire way of thinking grew up around them.

The first is hydrogen, a primary byproduct of bacteria fermenting carbohydrates. It crosses into your blood, travels to your lungs, and gets exhaled, which is the whole basis of breath testing in the first place. A rise in exhaled hydrogen after you drink a sugar solution suggests bacteria in your small intestine are fermenting that sugar too early and too eagerly. The second is methane, produced by a specific group of microbes that consume hydrogen and make methane in its place, a pattern now often called intestinal methanogen overgrowth, or IMO, and strongly associated with constipation (Pimentel et al., 2020). Two gases. Two stories. For a long time that framework did real good, giving clinicians a way to tell apart patterns that had all previously been lumped together under the vague umbrella of irritable bowel syndrome.

But a two-gas test can only ever tell a two-gas story, and a great many people were living a third one. The third gas is hydrogen sulfide, and it is made by yet another group of organisms, the sulfate-reducing bacteria, which consume hydrogen and combine it with the sulfur available in the gut to produce hydrogen sulfide gas (Banaszak et al., 2023). In small amounts, hydrogen sulfide is normal and even useful. The problem is overproduction, when these bacteria proliferate and the gas they generate climbs beyond what the gut lining can comfortably handle. Because this gas can be produced throughout the gut rather than only in the small intestine, the more precise name gaining ground is intestinal sulfide overproduction, or ISO (Trio-Smart, 2023). I will use both terms in this book, because you will meet both in the wild, but ISO is where the language is heading.

This is where I want to plant the idea that does more work than any single fact in these pages. Hydrogen sulfide overgrowth is not a new disease that appeared out of nowhere. It is a newly measurable one. The people who have it were not imagining their symptoms during all the years the test could not see the gas responsible. They were waiting for the instruments, and the vocabulary, to catch up with what their bodies already knew.

Why the gas hides inside a normal result

Now for the mechanism that explains Ozias's clean second test, and possibly yours, because once you see it you cannot unsee it.

Remember that the sulfate-reducing bacteria make their gas by consuming hydrogen. Picture what that does to a hydrogen breath test. The fermenting bacteria produce hydrogen, yes, but the sulfate reducers consume it to build their sulfide, drawing it down almost as fast as it appears. The hydrogen never accumulates enough to register a clear rise. On the printout, the line stays low and flat. The methane line, if you are not a methane producer, stays flat too. Two flat lines, nothing crosses a threshold, and the report prints the word negative (Ruscio, 2024). The gas driving the symptoms was there the entire time. The test simply had no channel to record it, and worse, the very act of making that gas erased the one signal the test could have caught.

This is what I call, in the shorthand I use with people I work with, the Unmeasured Third. The principle is simple and worth holding onto: a standard breath test measures two gases and is silent about the third, so a normal result can hide a real overgrowth rather than rule one out. It is not that the test is useless. It is that the test answers only the questions it was built to ask, and a flat line, in the right body, is not a clean bill of health but a clue pointing straight at the subtype the machine could not measure.

Ozias sat with that for a moment when I explained it, the folder still open in front of him. Then he said something I have heard, in one form or another, from many people since. He said that for three years he had believed either the machine was broken or he was. And it turned out neither was true. The machine was working exactly as designed. It had simply been designed to look for two things, and his problem was the third. That reframe did not cure him. But it moved him, in a single conversation, from a man clutching a folder of evidence that no one would read to a man with a specific, nameable, addressable hypothesis about his own body. And that shift, from adrift to oriented, is where every recovery in this book begins.

We have laid the foundation. Overgrowth is a real, mechanical process. It produces different gases in different people. And the third gas, hydrogen sulfide, went unmeasured for years and hides inside results that look normal. What we have not yet done is learn to read that flat line properly, in a report and in a body, and that is exactly where we go next.

Chapter 2: Reading The Flat Line

Zae kept her breath test report folded into quarters in the front pocket of her bag, and by the time she showed it to me the creases had gone soft and furred from handling. She had read it, she guessed, several hundred times. Across the top it said, in the flat language laboratories use, that no significant rise in hydrogen or methane had been detected, and she had been told this meant she did not have SIBO. In the two years since, she had built a private theory that the machine had somehow failed her, because the only alternative she could see was that the paper was right and her suffering was invented, and that alternative she refused. She was right to refuse it. But she was chasing the wrong fix. She did not need a better theory about a broken machine. She needed somebody to teach her how to read the sheet already in her hands.

That is what this chapter does. Not to throw out the breath test, which is a genuinely useful tool, but to understand exactly what it can and cannot tell you, and to recognize the one pattern that gets mislabeled as nothing more often than any other.

What the test is actually doing

The breath test is elegant and limited in equal measure, and you need to hold both halves of that to use it well.

You arrive having fasted, having followed a preparation diet the day before. You drink a measured dose of a sugar that bacteria can ferment, usually lactulose or glucose. Then, over the next two to three hours, you breathe into a series of tubes at set intervals, and the gas in those tubes gets analyzed and plotted against time to make a curve (Rezaie et al., 2017). The logic is that if bacteria are overgrown up in the small intestine, they will reach the sugar early, ferment it early, and produce a detectable rise in gas well before that sugar would normally arrive down in the large intestine. A rise in hydrogen crossing an agreed line within that early window reads as consistent with hydrogen overgrowth. A rise in methane, which tends to run flatter and higher across the whole test, points toward the methane pattern (Rezaie et al., 2017).

And there it is, tucked into that description, the thing that changes everything for a person holding a normal result. The test measures hydrogen and methane. It measures what it measures, and it says nothing about anything else. A great deal of unnecessary despair flows from forgetting that a test can only ever report on the questions it was built to ask. Zae had spent two years treating a two-gas answer as if it were a verdict on her whole gut. It was never that. It was an answer to two specific questions, and her problem was a third question the test had not asked.

The shape of a flat line

Of all the patterns a breath test can throw, the flat line is the one most likely to be waved away, and the one most worth a second look.

A flat line is exactly what it sounds like. Across the whole test, neither hydrogen nor methane climbs in any meaningful way. The curves stay low and level from the first tube to the last. Because nothing crosses a threshold, the report generates as negative, and in a lot of settings that is where the conversation ends (Ruscio, 2024). Now, honesty requires me to tell you that a flat line can mean more than one thing. Occasionally it reflects a genuinely quiet gut with no overgrowth at all. Occasionally it reflects a technical problem, a sample that was not deep lung air, or a rare person whose flora simply does not make much hydrogen. Those possibilities are real and I will not pretend otherwise.

But there is one more possibility, and it is the one standard interpretation routinely leaves out. The flat line may mean that hydrogen is being produced and then eaten before it can build up. If a population of sulfate-reducing bacteria is drawing hydrogen down to manufacture hydrogen sulfide, the hydrogen curve can be flattened into silence even while fermentation is going full tilt (Ruscio, 2024). The process causing the symptoms erases the signal that would have revealed it. Read that way, a flat line is not the absence of a problem. It can be the fingerprint of the one gas the test could not see.

This is the principle I want you to carry out of this chapter, and I call it the Silent Flat Line: a flat breath test in a person full of symptoms is not a clearance but a clue, because the sulfide subtype suppresses the very hydrogen the test relies on. Say it to yourself the next time you look at that word negative. It is not the end of the sentence. It may be the beginning of the real one.

Why suppression looks like silence

It is worth slowing down on the mechanism, because once it clicks it becomes a permanent tool you carry for reading any report of this kind.

Picture two teams of microbes sharing your small intestine. The first team ferments the sugar you drank and pumps out hydrogen. Ordinarily that hydrogen builds up, crosses into your blood, reaches your lungs, and shows up on the test as a rising curve. But the second team, the sulfate reducers, treats hydrogen as fuel. They eat it as fast as it appears and combine it with sulfur to make hydrogen sulfide. The hydrogen never gets the chance to accumulate. On the printout, the first team's work is invisible, hidden by the second team's appetite, and the gas the second team makes has no line of its own on a two-gas test. The result is a report that says quiet when your gut is anything but.

Timing adds a wrinkle worth knowing. A suppression that shows up in the later part of the test, as the sugar reaches the far end of the small intestine, has drawn particular interest as a marker worth taking seriously, though the field is still working out exactly how much weight to give it. None of this means every flat line is hydrogen sulfide. It means a flat line in the wrong body, next to the wrong symptoms, deserves investigation rather than dismissal. The gap between those two responses is often the gap between a person who finally gets answers and a person who spends another two years with a soft-creased sheet folded into the pocket of a bag.

When you cannot get the newer test

You may be wondering whether a test exists that can see the third gas directly, and the answer is yes, with real qualifications. Breath testing that measures hydrogen sulfide directly has become available in recent years, giving the gas its own line at last rather than leaving it to be inferred (Trio-Smart, 2023). Where you can get it and afford it, it can turn a years-long guessing game into a measured result. But it is not available everywhere, access and cost vary enormously, and like any test it must be prepared for and read correctly, because a poorly prepared test misleads no matter how many gases it counts.

So a great many readers will want the newer test and be unable to get it, and I refuse to leave you stranded there, because you are not stranded. Long before direct sulfide testing existed, clinicians recognized and worked with this pattern using what is called an empiric approach, meaning a diagnosis reasoned from the whole picture rather than confirmed by a single number (Ruscio, 2024). The pieces of that picture are the ones this book is handing you. A flat-line result. A symptom pattern that fits the sulfide type, which the next chapter details. And a clear response to a deliberate reduction in dietary sulfur. When those three line up, a reasonable clinician can proceed on the working idea of sulfide overgrowth without a confirmatory number, adjusting as the evidence comes in.

Lorcan lived somewhere he could not get three-gas testing at all. His clinician looked at his flat-line report, took a careful history, and suggested a structured trial of reduced sulfur for a set period. His symptoms eased noticeably within a couple of weeks and came back when he reintroduced high-sulfur foods too fast. That pattern, taken together, told them something no single test could have. It was not a laboratory-stamped diagnosis, and his clinician said so plainly. But it was enough to justify a direction, which for Lorcan beat the dead end he had been staring at for a year. Carry the reframe forward. The breath test is a tool, not a verdict, a flat line is a clue, not a clearance, and the person who cannot get the newest test can still read the pattern from the fuller picture. We turn now to the body itself, and to the symptoms that, understood correctly, are the strongest evidence you carry.

Chapter 3: Beyond The Rotten Egg

Morag had ruled herself out, and she had done it years earlier, on the strength of a single fact she had read in passing.

She had every reason to suspect her gut. Relentless bloating, a fatigue that sleep never touched, a stomach that inflated after meals she could not predict. At some point she had read that hydrogen sulfide SIBO smells of rotten eggs, and her gas did not smell of rotten eggs, not that she had noticed, and so she had crossed the sulfide subtype off her list and gone on searching elsewhere, or, more accurately, had mostly stopped searching, because the elsewhere had run out. When she finally landed in front of a clinician who took her flat-line test, her bloating, her fatigue, and her striking reactions to garlic and eggs seriously, the sulfide idea came back onto the table, and it fit almost everything. The one thing that had kept her from it for years was a smell she did not have, and, as it turned out, did not need.

Her mistake is the single most common one people make with this condition, and this chapter exists to dismantle it, because the true shape of the sulfide pattern is broader, stranger, and more forgiving than the rotten-egg caricature allows.

The smell that misleads

The famous symptom is real. Hydrogen sulfide smells of rotten eggs, and when it is produced in excess in the gut, the gas and the belches that come with it can carry that smell unmistakably. For some people it is the most socially distressing part of the whole condition, a symptom that reshapes where they will eat and whom they will sit beside. I am not going to tell you the smell is a myth, because it is not.

What is a myth is the belief that grew up around it, the assumption that no rotten-egg smell means no hydrogen sulfide problem. That assumption is wrong, and clinical descriptions of the condition increasingly say so outright, that the characteristic odor is variable and not required for the diagnosis (Lindemann, 2026). Plenty of people with genuine sulfide overgrowth never notice a strong sulfur smell, or notice it only sometimes, or have simply lived with it so long they no longer register it as remarkable. The danger is in what people do with the belief. They experience relentless gut symptoms, read that the condition smells of rotten eggs, notice no such smell, and conclude the sulfide subtype cannot be theirs. They cross it off, exactly as Morag did.

So here is the principle, and I call it the Missing Smell: the rotten-egg odor is a clue when it is present and means nothing at all when it is absent, so its absence must never be used to rule the condition out. The smell can point toward sulfide. It can never point away from it. A person who has excluded themselves because their gas does not smell of eggs has excluded themselves on no evidence whatsoever, and they deserve to put themselves back on the list.

The fuller cluster

Take the fixation on smell away and a richer, more useful picture comes into focus, drawn from how the condition actually shows up across large groups of people.

The most common complaints are not exotic. Bloating leads by a wide margin, followed by abdominal pain, fatigue, flatulence, and altered bowel habits (Nutrition Resolution, 2026). On their own these could describe almost any gut disorder, which is precisely why sulfide overgrowth hides so well inside the broad label of irritable bowel syndrome. It is the extra, less obvious features that begin to set it apart. Alongside the core gut symptoms, clinicians who work with this condition report a wider cluster that patients themselves rarely connect to their gut: sulfur-smelling gas or burps when present, skin complaints, urinary symptoms, odd neurological sensations such as tingling, a vague but insistent sense of feeling toxic or unwell, heightened sensitivity to light or sound, and, very tellingly, adverse reactions to high-sulfur foods and to sulfur-containing supplements.

No single one of these confirms anything. Together, layered over the core gut picture, they begin to form a recognizable silhouette. The lesson is not that you should tally these symptoms and diagnose yourself, which no book can responsibly help you do. The lesson is that the sulfide pattern is a whole-body pattern more often than people expect, and that symptoms which seem to have nothing to do with digestion may belong to the same story. Recognizing that can be the moment a scattered set of complaints resolves into a single, addressable hypothesis, which is what happened for Morag once someone helped her see the shape of it.

The constipation nobody warns you about

If the rotten-egg myth is the first thing that wrongly excludes people, the diarrhea myth is the second, and it is just as important to take apart.

The common teaching pairs hydrogen sulfide with diarrhea, and there is a basis for it, since higher sulfide levels do correlate with looser, more urgent stools in many people, and the association is real (Nutrition Resolution, 2026). But it has hardened into an overstatement that leaves a whole subgroup of sufferers convinced they cannot possibly have the condition. When large groups of diagnosed sulfide patients are actually examined, constipation turns up nearly as often as diarrhea, and mixed patterns, alternating between the two, are common as well. Morag's dominant symptom was constipation so stubborn that she had assumed her problem was purely a motility issue with no connection to any overgrowth. She had read repeatedly that sulfide meant diarrhea, and since diarrhea was not her experience, she had set the whole idea aside. Her case was not a rare exception. It was an ordinary presentation that the tidy diarrhea rule had hidden from her.

Hold both corrections together, because between them they rescue an enormous number of people. The smell may be absent. The bowel pattern may be constipation, diarrhea, or a mixture of the two. Neither the missing smell nor the constipation rules out sulfide overgrowth, and a person who has written themselves off on either ground has written themselves off too soon.

Building your own picture

There is one more feature of this condition worth naming, because it sends so many people down the wrong path, and that is the way it produces symptoms that do not feel like gut symptoms at all. Fatigue out of all proportion to sleep. Brain fog, a sense of thinking through fabric. Because these do not look digestive, they often get chased down entirely separate roads, investigated as thyroid problems or mood disorders while the gut process quietly driving them goes unexamined. The mechanism is not fully mapped, and I would rather admit that than invent a tidy story, but the pattern is clinically clear enough that experienced clinicians look for these systemic symptoms, and their presence alongside the gut picture strengthens rather than muddies the case.

Which brings us to the real work of this chapter, which is not a diagnosis but a description, because the ability to describe your own pattern accurately turns out to be one of the most valuable things you can bring to a clinician. Most people arrive at appointments with a vague, apologetic account, and vagueness invites dismissal. A person who can say plainly that they have persistent bloating, mixed bowel habits, an unshakable fatigue, a flat-line breath test, and a reliable worsening after eggs and garlic is handing their clinician a coherent hypothesis instead of a shrug. So over the coming days, notice your pattern without judging it. Notice which symptoms cluster and when they worsen. Notice whether the smell is present, absent, or intermittent, and refuse to draw any conclusion from its absence. Notice your bowel pattern honestly, whichever way it runs, and record the fatigue and the fog even though they do not feel like they belong. You are assembling the strongest line of evidence you carry, the one no laboratory can produce for you. With the test read correctly and the symptoms seen clearly, we are ready for the most confusing part of this whole subject, the tangle of words around sulfur itself.

Chapter 4: The Sulfur Confusion

Phaedon showed me his list of everything he had given up, and it was long, and almost none of it was helping, and the reason it was not helping is the reason this chapter exists.

He had been at it for months. He had stopped drinking wine because of the sulfites. He had thrown out his dried apricots for the same reason. He had switched to a special shampoo without sulfates. He had stopped taking Epsom salt baths. He had swapped his mineral water for a brand with less sulfate in it. He was, by his own account, being enormously disciplined, and he was proud of it, and he was also no better than when he started. Because while he was policing all of that, he was still eating eggs at breakfast and cooking nearly everything in garlic, and nobody had helped him see that these, not the apricots or the bathwater, were the things actually feeding his problem. He had waged a long, exhausting campaign against the wrong enemy, and the right enemy had been on his plate the whole time.

This happens constantly, and it is not the fault of the people it happens to. It happens because several different things share a similar name, and a great deal of writing on this subject blurs them together, manufacturing fear where there should be clarity and offering none where there should be caution.

Four words that are not the same

The words that cause all the trouble are sulfur, sulfite, sulfate, and thiol. They sound like relatives, and chemically they are cousins, but for a person with hydrogen sulfide overgrowth they behave completely differently and demand completely different responses.

Sulfur, in the sense that matters here, means chiefly the sulfur in certain amino acids, the building blocks of protein, and in particular compounds in some vegetables. This is the sulfur that sulfate-reducing bacteria draw on to make hydrogen sulfide. When this book talks about reducing sulfur, this is overwhelmingly what it means. Sulfites are something else entirely. They are preservatives, added to wine, dried fruit, and processed foods to stop spoilage. Some people are sensitive to sulfites, but that sensitivity usually shows up as respiratory symptoms, asthma-like reactions most notably, rather than as the gut problem we are discussing (Bryan, 2021). Sulfite sensitivity and hydrogen sulfide overgrowth are separate issues that happen to share a syllable.

Sulfates are sulfur bound to oxygen, found in mineral waters, in Epsom salts, in some medications. Thiols are sulfur-containing compounds present in certain foods and central to some supplements. Each of these can matter in specific circumstances, but each is its own category, and treating all four as a single enemy, which is exactly what Phaedon had done, is the surest route to a diet that is both needlessly restrictive and aimed at the wrong target.

Why the confusion sticks around

It is worth understanding why so much published material muddles these categories, because seeing where the confusion comes from helps protect you from it.

Part of the problem is that the writing on this subject has outrun the science that should anchor it. As interest in the sulfide subtype grew, a flood of consumer content appeared, much of it assembled quickly by borrowing from neighboring topics. Advice written for people with sulfite asthma got imported wholesale into guidance for people with gut sulfide overgrowth, and the two got tangled (Bryan, 2021). Advice about thiols, some of it drawn from contexts that concern the bloodstream rather than the gut, got folded in too, even though the relevance of thiol restriction to intestinal sulfide production is far less established than the confident tone of some sources suggests. The result is guidance in which a single article warns you off wine and dried fruit and Epsom salts and shampoo and a long list of foods, as though all of them fed the same fire. They do not.

This is why the competitor books on this subject so often fail their readers. They inherit the confusion instead of resolving it, and they pass it on intact. A reader who cannot tell sulfur from sulfite from sulfate cannot build a sensible plan, because they do not know which thing they are meant to be reducing. Which gives us the principle for this chapter, and I call it the Four Sulfur Words: sulfur, sulfite, sulfate, and thiol are distinct, and only dietary sulfur is the central lever for gut sulfide overgrowth, so lumping them together wastes effort on the wrong things.

What actually matters for your gut

Cut through all of it and the practical center of gravity is narrower and far more manageable than the fear-laden lists suggest.

For most people with this condition, the dietary levers that matter are the sulfur-containing amino acids in protein and the sulfur compounds in a specific set of vegetables, above all the allium family, meaning garlic, onions, leeks, and their relatives, and the cruciferous family, meaning broccoli, cabbage, cauliflower, and kale. Eggs, rich in sulfur amino acids, are a frequent trigger. These are the foods whose reduction most reliably calms sulfide production (Nutrition Resolution, 2026). Notice what is not on that central list. Sulfite preservatives in wine and dried fruit are not, for most gut sulfide sufferers, the main issue, though a person who separately has sulfite sensitivity has their own reasons for care. Sulfate in an Epsom salt bath is not being eaten. The sulfate in a shampoo is not entering your small intestine. Many medications containing sulfate compounds are not the target either, and no one should stop a prescribed medication over sulfur fears without speaking to the prescriber.

This narrowing is a relief, and it is meant to be. So much of the anxiety around this condition comes from an unbounded sense that sulfur is everywhere and must be hunted down in every corner of a life. It is not, and it does not. The battlefield is smaller and better defined than the panic suggests.

A simple way to decide

Because the categories are easy to relearn and easy to forget, carry a simple rule you can apply to anything that provokes uncertainty. Ask first whether you are eating the item, because if it is not being eaten, it is almost never relevant to gut sulfide production, and a bath additive or a shampoo falls away immediately. Ask second, of the things you eat, whether the item is a real source of sulfur amino acids or of allium or cruciferous sulfur, because those are the sources that feed the process. Ask third whether your own experience confirms a reaction, because individual tolerance varies enormously and your body's response is better evidence than any list.

Run Phaedon through those three questions and his whole approach rearranges itself. The apricots, the bathwater, the mineral water fall away under the first question, which lifts a real weight. The eggs and the garlic light up under the second and, once he looked honestly, the third. He stopped policing the irrelevant things and redirected his attention to the foods his own reactions confirmed were the problem, and only then did his symptoms begin to move. That is the whole point of this chapter. Not more restriction, but better-aimed restriction. The tangle of sulfur words has cost readers an enormous amount of pointless avoidance and an enormous amount of missed opportunity, and cutting through it lets you spend your effort where it counts. With the vocabulary finally clear, we can meet the organisms at the heart of all this, and ask why they overgrew in you in the first place.

Chapter 5: The Bacteria Behind It

Cashel could name the week his gut broke, though he did not realize it was the week until we went looking for it together.

He had come in convinced his overgrowth had appeared from nowhere, one of those things that just happens to a body for no reason. But as we walked backward through his history, a moment surfaced. Several years earlier, on a trip abroad, he had come down with a severe stomach illness, the kind that empties you out for the better part of a week and then, apparently, passes. He had filed it away as an unpleasant episode long resolved. What it had actually left behind was a subtly damaged cleaning system in his gut, and on that damaged ground, slowly, an overgrowth had established itself. Naming that week did not undo it, and I was honest with him that this kind of damage is not always fully reversible. But it reframed everything about his treatment, because it explained why every attempt to simply kill the bacteria had kept failing him.

This chapter is about the organisms behind hydrogen sulfide overgrowth, but more than that, it is about the ground they grew on, because the ground is the part almost everyone misses, and missing it is why so many people relapse.

Meet the sulfate reducers

The organisms responsible for hydrogen sulfide overproduction are called sulfate-reducing bacteria, and their name describes exactly what they do. They make their living by taking sulfate and other sulfur compounds and reducing them, in the chemical sense, using hydrogen as fuel, and the waste product of that metabolism is hydrogen sulfide gas (Achufusi et al., 2020). In an ordinary gut, in ordinary numbers, they are just part of the crowd, and the small amounts of sulfide they make are handled comfortably by the gut lining, which even puts hydrogen sulfide to legitimate use. The problem, as with all overgrowth, is one of quantity and location, not of the mere presence of the organism.

Certain names recur in the research, and you may run into them. Desulfovibrio is the one most often tied to intestinal hydrogen sulfide, and its abundance has been linked to sulfide-related gut trouble in several lines of investigation (Achufusi et al., 2020). Other organisms take part too. I mention these not so you can hunt for them on a stool test and panic at their presence, because they live in healthy guts as well, but so the vocabulary is familiar if it appears and the process feels concrete rather than mysterious. And I want to plant a reframe right here, because it changes how you will hear everything about treatment later. The goal is not to sterilize your gut. A gut with no sulfate-reducing bacteria at all is neither achievable nor desirable. The goal is to bring an overgrown population back into proportion, which is a very different and far more humane aim than waging chemical war on your own insides.

The hydrogen connection

There is a reason hydrogen sulfide overgrowth so often travels alongside the older, better-known hydrogen subtype, and it explains a great deal of otherwise baffling experience.

Remember that sulfate reducers use hydrogen as fuel, and that hydrogen has to come from somewhere. Where it comes from is the fermentation carried out by other bacteria, the same fermentation that defines classic hydrogen overgrowth. The two processes are linked. Fermenters make hydrogen, sulfate reducers eat it, and so the two populations tend to rise and fall together and often share the same gut (Achufusi et al., 2020). This is not a curiosity. It is the reason a person can be treated for hydrogen overgrowth, improve, and then relapse, because the sulfide-producing partners were never addressed and carried on once the treatment pressure lifted. It also explains that maddening pattern of the person who tests positive for hydrogen, gets treated, and improves only partway, their fermenters knocked back while their sulfate reducers, feeding on whatever hydrogen remained, kept going. To that person the treatment looks like a partial success that mysteriously stalls, when in truth it addressed one member of a two-member partnership and left the other in place.

Why they overgrew in you

Now the most important question in this chapter, and also the one most often skipped, which is why so many people relapse. The question is not what organisms are overgrown, but why they were able to overgrow in the first place.

Overgrowth is rarely random. It happens when the gut's housekeeping falters and bacteria pile up where they should be swept clear. The most common culprit is impaired motility, and in particular a weakened version of that between-meal cleaning wave (Deloose et al., 2012). A frequent cause of that weakening is exactly what happened to Cashel, a prior bout of gastroenteritis, a case of food poisoning or a stomach bug, that damages the nerves governing gut motility and leaves behind a small intestine that no longer cleans itself efficiently. This is one of the best-established routes into SIBO of any kind. Other drivers populate the list too. Low stomach acid removes a barrier that would otherwise limit bacterial survival. Structural quirks create pockets where bacteria stagnate. Certain medications and prior surgeries alter the terrain. And chronic stress, through its well-documented effects on gut function, can tilt the balance over time. No single one of these is the cause. Each is a way the gut's defenses can be lowered enough for overgrowth to take hold.

This gives us the principle for this chapter, the one Cashel's story is built to teach, and I call it the Terrain Beneath: bacteria overgrow because the ground allowed it, so any lasting recovery has to address the ground and not only the bacteria.

Why killing bacteria is not enough

Here is the reframe this whole chapter has been building toward. The intuitive model of overgrowth is a military one. Bacteria have invaded, so you kill them, and the problem is solved. If that model were right, a single course of treatment would reliably end the matter for most people. It does not, and the reason is that the military model leaves out the terrain. If the conditions that allowed the overgrowth remain unchanged, the impaired motility, the lowered defenses, the underlying driver, then reducing the bacterial population simply clears space for it to grow back. You can win the battle and lose the war, over and over, wondering why the enemy keeps returning.

This is not an argument against treatment, which has a real and important place, taken up in a later chapter. It is an argument against treatment in isolation. The durable approach pairs any effort to reduce the overgrown population with equal attention to the ground that permitted it, supporting motility, addressing the driver where it can be addressed, removing the conditions that favor regrowth (Deloose et al., 2012). This is unglamorous work, and it lacks the satisfying decisiveness of a kill-and-cure, which is exactly why it gets neglected in favor of repeated rounds of antimicrobials that keep almost working. So the exercise this chapter leaves you with is reflection rather than action. Look back across your own history and ask what might have lowered your gut's defenses. Was there a bout of food poisoning or a stomach bug before your troubles began, as there was for Cashel? A stretch of high stress, a surgery, a long course of a medication that reduces stomach acid? You may not find one clean answer, and that is fine. But identifying a plausible driver, where one exists, reshapes everything that follows, because it turns treatment from repeated demolition into genuine repair. With the organisms understood and the ground examined, we can take up the intervention people most associate with this condition, and do it properly, which means doing it as a tool rather than a sentence.

Chapter 6: The Low Sulfur Diet

Delyth did the low-sulfur diet so well that it nearly hurt her, and her story is the reason I put a warning at the front of this chapter instead of the back.

She was thorough by nature, and when she read that protein was high in sulfur, she did the thorough thing. She cut it to almost nothing. For weeks she lived on rice and a short list of low-sulfur vegetables, and her bloating did ease somewhat, which she took as proof she was on the right track. But she grew exhausted in a way that went beyond her usual fatigue. She lost weight she could not afford to lose. She started feeling faint on the stairs. When her clinician finally saw what her diet had become, the alarm was immediate, because Delyth had not been treating her gut. She had been slowly starving herself in pursuit of a symptom, and the diet's poor framing had invited her to do it. Her first attempt was not a failure of discipline. It was a mistake that better guidance would have prevented, and preventing it for you is a large part of why this chapter is written the way it is.

The low-sulfur diet is the most useful dietary tool for calming hydrogen sulfide overgrowth. It is also, in the wrong framing, a route into months of fearful, self-punishing restriction that harms the person more than the overgrowth ever did. Both of those are true at once, and the framing you bring decides which one you get.

A tool, not a sentence

Before a single food is named, the most important sentence in this chapter has to be said plainly. The low-sulfur diet is a temporary tool with a defined purpose and a planned end, not a way of eating you are meant to adopt for life.

Its purpose is twofold. First, it is diagnostic. A clear improvement when sulfur is reduced, and a clear return of symptoms when it comes back, is meaningful evidence pointing toward sulfide overgrowth, and it is especially valuable for the many people who cannot get direct testing (Nutrition Resolution, 2026). Second, it is calming. By lowering the raw material available to sulfate-reducing bacteria, it can reduce sulfide production and give a distressed gut some relief while the rest of a plan does its work. Neither purpose requires, or benefits from, going on forever. The clinician whose framing I trust most describes the low-sulfur diet not as the solution but as the clue that points toward the solution, and insists thc goal is always to widen the diet back out rather than narrow it forever (Nutrition Resolution, 2026).

That gives us the principle for this chapter, and I call it the Borrowed Diet: the low-sulfur diet is borrowed for a short, defined stretch to gather information and buy relief, and it must always be given back. A food list in the hands of a frightened person with no exit plan becomes a cage. The same list, held as a short experiment with a scheduled review and a reintroduction to follow, becomes a genuinely useful instrument. The list is identical. The framing is everything.

Understanding the tiers

With the framing in place, the food landscape becomes navigable, and it is best understood not as a wall between forbidden and permitted but as a set of tiers.

At the high-sulfur end sit the foods most worth reducing during a trial, the sulfur-rich proteins, especially eggs, and among plants the allium family of garlic, onions, and leeks and the cruciferous family of broccoli, cauliflower, cabbage, and kale (Nutrition Resolution, 2026). These are not poisons. They are healthy foods in an ordinary diet. They are simply the richest sources of the sulfur that feeds the process, which is exactly why a person with sulfide overgrowth so often reacts to them. In the middle sit foods of moderate sulfur content that many people tolerate in reasonable portions and need not eliminate wholesale. And at the low end sit the foods that form the backbone of a workable trial, including many well-tolerated proteins in modest portions, rice, various squashes, and a range of lower-sulfur vegetables. The appendices carry a fuller tiered reference, because a list of that kind is more useful to consult than to read straight through.

Thinking in tiers rather than absolutes protects you from the all-or-nothing thinking that makes these diets so miserable. You are not dividing the world into safe and forbidden. You are lowering your overall sulfur load for a defined period, leaning toward the lower tiers, easing off the highest ones, and watching what your body does.

The protein problem

No part of this diet causes more quiet harm than the handling of protein, because the obvious move is the wrong one, and Delyth made it.

The difficulty is real. The sulfur-containing amino acids are in all animal protein, which means the most sulfur-dense foods overlap heavily with the most important protein sources (Specialists in Gastroenterology, n.d.). Faced with that, the intuitive response is to slash protein, and a lot of people do exactly what Delyth did and end up weak, hungry, losing muscle, and no better in the gut, because under-eating protein is genuinely harmful and does not even target the problem precisely. The better approach is to reduce sulfur load rather than abandon protein, and load is a function of three things, the type of protein, the portion size, and the timing. Choosing lower-sulfur sources where you can, keeping portions moderate rather than enormous, and spreading protein across the day rather than stacking it can all lower the sulfur burden while keeping intake adequate (Specialists in Gastroenterology, n.d.). Adequate is the word to hold onto. You need enough protein to maintain your body, and cutting below that to chase a gut symptom trades one problem for a worse one. Delyth's clinician rebuilt her plan around moderate portions of better-tolerated protein spread through the day, and the result was a gut nearly as calm as before but a body no longer starving.

Running a proper trial

A low-sulfur diet undertaken vaguely and indefinitely teaches you little and costs you a great deal. Run as a structured trial, it teaches you a great deal and costs you little, and the whole difference is structure.

A proper trial has a defined length, commonly two to four weeks, long enough to reveal a response but short enough not to drift into open-ended restriction (Nutrition Resolution, 2026). It has a clear method, leaning toward the lower tiers while keeping protein adequate. And it has measurement, a simple daily record of your main symptoms scored the same way each day, so you are reading data rather than trusting the unreliable impression of whether you feel better. The appendices give you a template for exactly this, because memory is a poor instrument for tracking gradual change. At the end of the period, you read the result honestly. A clear, meaningful easing of symptoms points toward sulfur as a genuine driver and justifies moving into the later stages of a plan, including the reintroduction a later chapter details. An ambiguous or absent response is also informative, since it suggests sulfur may not be your primary lever and the search should turn elsewhere rather than deeper into restriction.

I want to close with the warnings, because a diet chapter without them would be irresponsible, and because Delyth is the reason I know they matter. Stop the trial and seek help if you are losing weight you did not mean to lose, if faintness or weakness sets in, or if the restriction begins to feed fear or a sense of losing control around food. These are not signs to push through. They are signs the tool has become the problem, and no gut symptom is worth trading for that. If you have any history of disordered eating, do not run this trial alone at all, but work through it with a clinician or a registered dietitian who can hold the framing steady when you cannot. The diet is a means to a wider life, never an end in itself, and the moment it stops serving that end, it should be set down.

Chapter 7: When Healthy Foods Backfire

Ephie had cleaned up her diet, and cleaning up her diet was making her sick, and she had almost convinced herself she was imagining the whole thing because the food was, by every standard she knew, beyond reproach.

When her gut symptoms worsened, she had done what a conscientious person does. She loaded her plates with the foods everyone praises. Eggs for protein at breakfast. Garlic and onions in nearly every dinner because they are supposed to be good for you. Broccoli, cauliflower, kale, the whole celebrated roster of cruciferous vegetables. The healthier her diet looked on paper, the worse she felt in her body, and the contradiction was so sharp that she began to suspect her symptoms were psychological, because surely the food could not be the problem. The food was not the problem in any general sense. It was the problem for her particular gut, and once she understood that her impeccable diet was, from a sulfur standpoint, close to worst-case, and eased off the highest-sulfur items, the improvement was so rapid it was almost disorienting, because it overturned an assumption she had built her entire approach on.

This chapter is written for that bewilderment, the specific vertigo of a body that rebels against the very things it was told would heal it. The explanation is not that you are broken. It is that in a gut prone to sulfide overproduction, some of the healthiest-sounding foods and supplements are exactly the ones that feed the fire.

The supplement trap

The most dramatic version of this involves supplements, because supplements deliver concentrated doses of compounds that food never would, and several of the most fashionable ones are essentially sulfur in a capsule.

The names to know are N-acetylcysteine, usually written NAC, glutathione, and methylsulfonylmethane, usually written MSM. All three are sulfur-containing, and all three are marketed heavily for gut health, detoxification, and general wellness, which is precisely what makes them such a trap (Walsh, 2025). To a person with sulfide overgrowth, taking these can be like pouring fuel on the process, supplying the sulfur that sulfate-reducing bacteria turn into more of the gas driving their symptoms. The cruel irony is that these are often the very supplements a person reaches for in an effort to heal their gut, so the attempt to get better actively makes things worse.

Anhad found this out the hard way. In a determined push to fix his digestion, he assembled a stack of gut-healing supplements that included both NAC and glutathione, taken faithfully every morning. His symptoms, already troublesome, worsened sharply over the following weeks, and, reading that worsening as a sign he needed to try harder, he added more supplements, digging the hole deeper. It was only when a clinician reviewed his regimen and recognized the sulfur-heavy supplements for what they were that the picture came clear. Within days of stopping them, he improved. He had not been failing to heal for lack of effort. His effort had been aimed, through no fault of his own, directly at the wrong target. The lesson is not that these supplements are bad, since in other contexts they have legitimate uses. The lesson is the principle I call the Healthy Trap: a food or supplement being widely called healthy tells you nothing about whether it is right for your gut, and several of the most praised ones are common sulfide triggers.

The foods that turn on you

Beyond supplements, a familiar set of foods produces the same backfiring effect, and they are, frustratingly, some of the most celebrated foods in ordinary healthy eating.

Eggs are among the most common triggers, dense in sulfur amino acids. Garlic and onions, staples of good cooking and praised for their own health properties, are rich in allium sulfur and reliably provoke symptoms in many sulfide sufferers. The cruciferous vegetables, broccoli and cauliflower and cabbage and kale, celebrated as nutritional powerhouses, are significant sulfur sources too (Nutrition Resolution, 2026). A person who has dutifully built their diet around these foods, believing themselves to be eating impeccably, may be feeding their overgrowth several times a day, exactly as Ephie was. None of this makes these foods bad in any general sense, and I want to stress that so this chapter does not curdle into food fear. For most people, eggs and garlic and broccoli are exactly as healthy as their reputation. It is only in the specific context of sulfide overgrowth, and only for the duration that matters, that they warrant reduction, and the aim is always to return to them where tolerance allows.

Auditing your own intake

Because the triggers are so counterintuitive, the single most useful practical step is a deliberate audit of what you are actually consuming, since most people badly underestimate their sulfur load.

The exercise is simple. Over a few ordinary days, write down everything you eat and every supplement you take, without changing anything yet, because the goal at this stage is an honest picture rather than an intervention. Then go through the record and mark the high-sulfur items, the eggs, the alliums, the cruciferous vegetables, the large protein portions, and crucially the sulfur-containing supplements, the NAC and glutathione and MSM and anything similar (Walsh, 2025). Most people are startled by how much accumulates once they look, because sulfur-dense foods and popular supplements are so woven into what passes for healthy eating that their quantity goes unnoticed. The appendices provide a worksheet for this, and it is worth doing on paper rather than in your head, because the written version reveals patterns the mental version hides. What the audit gives you is a target list, not a list of foods to fear forever, but a set of specific, identified items to trial removing during the structured low-sulfur period, so you can see which of them your body actually reacts to.

Doing this without fear

A chapter about foods that backfire carries an obvious hazard, that it will leave you afraid of eating, and that outcome would be a failure of the whole thing, so I want to address it head-on. The purpose of identifying triggers is not to lengthen the list of things you fear. It is to give you information that reduces fear by replacing a vague dread of all food with a specific understanding of a limited set of items, tested and personal to you. Fear thrives on vagueness, on the sense that anything might be the problem and nothing is safe. Knowledge dissolves that. A person who knows that eggs and garlic are their triggers, confirmed by their own careful trial, is far freer than a person who suspects everything and understands nothing.

So hold the frame this book keeps returning to. Reduction is temporary and targeted. The identified triggers are candidates for reintroduction later, not permanent exiles, and a full chapter ahead is devoted to bringing foods back. Your tolerance is likely to widen as the underlying overgrowth is addressed, so a food that provokes symptoms now may be perfectly comfortable in time. And your own experience, gathered through honest observation, is more trustworthy than any generic list. The foods that backfire are not evidence that your body has turned against you. They are clues, specific and identifiable, and clues are the opposite of a mystery. With the diet understood as a tool and the triggers understood as information, we can turn to the harder practical question of how to get a real answer from a medical system that may never have heard of the condition you are learning to describe.

Chapter 8: Getting A Real Answer

Tovey had been dismissed twice before he learned that the problem was not only what he was saying but how he was saying it.

The first two appointments had gone the way so many of these appointments go. He had arrived anxious, talked in a long, apologetic loop about feeling unwell, watched the clinician's attention slide away, and left with nothing. By the third, something had changed, and the thing that had changed was preparation. He walked in with a single typed paragraph that summarized his flat-line test, his symptom cluster, and his clear response to reducing sulfur, along with three written questions. The encounter was completely different, not because his clinician was a different person, but because Tovey had handed her something concrete to engage with rather than a fog to wave away. She read the paragraph, considered the pattern, and agreed to pursue it. His preparation had not guaranteed the outcome, and he knew going in that it might not, but it had transformed the odds.

That is what this chapter is about. Not outsmarting your clinician or arriving armed for a fight, both of which backfire, but walking in prepared, describing your situation with a precision that invites investigation, and understanding the routes to an answer that stay open even when the newest test is out of reach.

The testing landscape, honestly

Before the conversation, it helps to know what testing can and cannot currently offer, because unrealistic expectations in either direction cause trouble.

The most direct route to confirmation is the breath test that measures hydrogen sulfide alongside hydrogen and methane, the three-gas test that gives sulfide its own line rather than leaving it to be inferred (Trio-Smart, 2023). Where it is available and affordable, it is the clearest single piece of evidence you can get, and it is reasonable to ask about it. But its availability is genuinely uneven, varying by country and health system and by whether local clinicians even know it exists, and it is not offered as a routine test in most standard settings. Ask about it without assuming it will be readily handed to you. Even the older two-gas test keeps its value here, because a flat-line result on it, as earlier chapters established, is itself a meaningful clue when read alongside the right symptoms (Ruscio, 2024). Many readers already hold such a result, dismissed as negative, and part of getting a real answer is bringing that result back into the conversation with a better interpretation attached.

Whatever test you pursue, preparation for it matters enormously and is worth raising with whoever administers it, because the day-before diet and the fasting window shape the result substantially, and a poorly prepared test misleads regardless of how many gases it counts.

When the test is not an option

For the substantial group who cannot get three-gas testing, the empiric route deserves real respect, because it is not a consolation prize but a legitimate, long-standing path.

An empiric approach reasons from the whole picture toward a working diagnosis, then uses the response to a careful intervention as further evidence (Ruscio, 2024). In this condition, that picture is assembled from the elements this book has been teaching, a flat-line result where one exists, a symptom cluster that fits the sulfide pattern, and a clear response to a deliberate, structured reduction in dietary sulfur. When those align, a reasonable clinician can proceed on the working hypothesis of sulfide overgrowth and adjust as the response unfolds, which is how a great deal of good medicine has always been practiced when a perfect test was not on offer. The response to the low-sulfur trial is particularly informative on this route, which is one more reason to run that trial as a proper structured experiment rather than a vague drift. A person who can report that their symptoms eased clearly during a defined low-sulfur period and returned when high-sulfur foods came back is offering a genuine piece of diagnostic evidence, gathered rigorously, that speaks directly to the sulfide question.

Preparing for the conversation

The encounter goes far better when you prepare, and preparation here means organizing what you know into a form a busy clinician can absorb quickly, because the sad truth is that dismissal often follows from disorganization as much as from ignorance.

The single most useful thing you can bring is the thing Tovey brought, a concise written summary of your situation, no more than a paragraph, stating your main symptoms, their duration, any test results you hold including a flat-line result, and any response you have observed to dietary changes (Achufusi et al., 2020). A clinician who receives a clear, specific account has something to reason about immediately. A clinician who receives a rambling, apologetic story has to do the organizing work themselves under time pressure, and that is exactly where good hypotheses get lost. The appendices provide a template for this summary, because writing it in advance, calmly, produces a far better document than trying to recall everything in the room. It also helps to bring your questions in writing, so anxiety in the moment does not erase them. Reasonable ones include whether three-gas testing is available or can be referred for, whether your flat-line result might fit the sulfide subtype, and whether a structured low-sulfur trial would be a sensible next step to pursue together. Framing these as questions you are exploring together, rather than demands or diagnoses you are asserting, tends to keep the clinician on your side, which is where you want them.

Which gives us the principle for this chapter, drawn straight from what changed between Tovey's second appointment and his third, and I call it the Prepared Paragraph: a single clear, specific written summary of your case does more to get you taken seriously than any amount of earnest explaining in the room.

When you are dismissed anyway

Preparation improves the odds but does not guarantee success, and honesty requires admitting that some readers, having done everything right, will still be dismissed, so this chapter has to address that rather than pretend it away.

If a clinician is genuinely unwilling to consider the sulfide subtype despite a well-prepared case, you have several reasonable options, and none of them is either surrender or hostility. You can seek a second opinion, ideally from a clinician with a known interest in gut disorders, since familiarity with this territory varies enormously between practitioners. You can seek out a registered dietitian with experience in SIBO, who may be both more accessible and more knowledgeable about the dietary approach than a general practitioner (Achufusi et al., 2020). And you can, within the bounds of safety, pursue the reasonable self-directed steps this book describes, chiefly the structured low-sulfur trial, which requires no prescription and generates exactly the kind of response evidence a future clinician will find persuasive. What you should not do is either give up on professional support or push into genuinely medical territory alone. The self-directed steps that are reasonable are dietary and observational. The steps that are not reasonable to take alone are the medical treatments the next chapter describes, which belong in the hands of a prescriber. Holding that line protects you, and it also strengthens your eventual case. Getting a real answer is a process you can influence, not a verdict handed down to you. You cannot control whether a given clinician takes you seriously, but you can control how clearly you describe your situation and how responsibly you pursue what is available to you, and those things genuinely move the odds. With the pursuit of an answer underway, we turn to the treatments themselves, which this book will describe so you can understand and discuss them, never so you can attempt them without the guidance they require.

Chapter 9: Your Treatment Options

Rune had been through two rounds of treatment aimed at killing his overgrowth, and each had helped for a while and then failed, and by the time I met him he had concluded that nothing worked and that he was simply one of the people medicine could not help.

He was wrong about that, but he was wrong in an understandable and instructive way. Both of his treatments had been aimed squarely at the bacteria, and both had knocked them back, and both times his symptoms had eased and then crept back over the following weeks. What neither treatment had touched was the impaired motility that kept letting the bacteria regrow, the ground beneath the whole problem. When he finally worked with a clinician who addressed that ground as well, supporting his motility and attending to his driver alongside a more considered reduction of the overgrowth, the result held in a way it never had before. Even then his clinician was careful to frame it as management requiring ongoing attention rather than a permanent cure. His earlier failures had not been evidence that he was untreatable. They had been evidence of an incomplete approach.

I have to put a warning on this chapter and mean it, because it runs through every paragraph. What follows is education, not instruction. It exists so you can understand the treatments used for hydrogen sulfide overgrowth and discuss them intelligently with a qualified prescriber, and for no other purpose. Nothing here is a protocol to follow, a dose to take, or a permission to treat yourself. Read this to become an informed participant in your own care. Do not read it as a manual, because it is not one.

The terrain behind treatment

Before any specific treatment makes sense, recall the lesson of Rune's story and of the chapter on bacteria, because it governs how the whole subject should be approached. Overgrowth is not merely a population of unwanted bacteria to be eliminated. It is a population that established itself because the gut's defenses were lowered, and any treatment aimed only at reducing the bacteria, while leaving the ground unchanged, invites regrowth (Deloose et al., 2012). This is why treatment of sulfide overgrowth is rarely a single decisive act and more often a combination of efforts, some aimed at reducing the overgrown population, some at supporting the motility and defenses that should keep it in check, and some at the dietary reduction that lowers the fuel supply. A prescriber thinking well about this holds all of these in view at once.

It is also why realistic expectations matter so much. A person hoping for one course of something that ends the matter forever is likely to be disappointed and to conclude, wrongly, that treatment does not work, which is exactly the trap Rune fell into. Treatment often works, but it works as part of a fuller approach and frequently requires iteration and attention to the ground, rather than functioning as a one-time cure. This gives us the principle for the chapter, and I call it the Informed Seat: your job is not to prescribe your own treatment but to occupy an informed seat at the table, understanding the options well enough to be a real participant in the decisions.

Reducing the overgrowth

The first category of treatment aims to reduce the overgrown population, and I discuss it only in the broadest educational terms, because the specifics belong to a prescriber.

One agent that recurs in discussions of hydrogen sulfide specifically is bismuth, familiar to many as the active ingredient in certain over-the-counter stomach remedies. Bismuth has a particular relevance here because research has shown it can reduce hydrogen sulfide in the gut, binding the gas in a way that addresses the sulfide problem somewhat distinctively compared with the other subtypes (Suarez et al., 1998). This is a real and interesting property, and it comes up often in the context of sulfide overgrowth. But whether, when, how, and for how long any bismuth-containing product should be used is a matter for a clinician, not for a reader, because even a familiar over-the-counter product carries considerations around dosing, duration, interactions, and individual suitability that require professional judgment. Beyond bismuth, treatment may involve antimicrobial approaches, whether herbal preparations or prescription antibiotics, chosen and directed by a clinician (Achufusi et al., 2020). I am deliberately not naming specific agents, doses, or regimens, because to do so would convert this educational discussion into exactly the protocol this chapter refuses to be. What matters for your understanding is that reducing the overgrowth is one arm of treatment, that several tools exist for it, and that the choice among them, and the manner of their use, is a clinical decision that depends on your particular situation.

Supporting the gut itself

The second category aims not at the bacteria but at the gut's own function, and it is the arm most often neglected, which is unfortunate, because it is frequently what makes the difference between a treatment that holds and one that fails, as Rune's story shows.

Central here is the support of motility, and in particular of that between-meal cleaning wave whose faltering so often permitted the overgrowth in the first place (Deloose et al., 2012). Approaches that support this wave, keeping the small intestine sweeping itself clear between meals, address the ground directly, and by doing so they can reduce the tendency to relapse that makes this condition so wearying. As with everything in this chapter, the specifics of which approach and how are a clinical matter, but the principle is worth understanding, because it explains why a prescriber may recommend ongoing support even after the acute overgrowth is reduced, and why abandoning that support the moment symptoms ease is such a common route back into trouble. Diet belongs in this supportive category too, in a role different from treatment proper. The low-sulfur reduction does not itself eliminate the overgrowth, but it lowers the fuel available to the sulfate-reducing bacteria and can calm symptoms while the other arms work (Nutrition Resolution, 2026). Held in its proper place, as a temporary calming measure rather than a cure, diet is a valuable part of the combination, and one of the few parts you can responsibly manage yourself, within the framing and cautions this book has stressed.

Being an informed participant

The purpose of this chapter, achieved or not, is to leave you able to participate in decisions about your treatment rather than merely receiving them, because informed participation produces better care and better adherence than passive compliance ever does.

An informed participant understands that treatment has these several arms and asks how they will be combined in their case. They understand that reducing the overgrowth without supporting the ground invites relapse, and can ask their clinician how the ground will be addressed. They understand that realistic timelines involve iteration rather than a single stroke, and are therefore less likely to abandon a working approach prematurely out of disappointment, as Rune nearly did. And they understand that even familiar over-the-counter products belong within a clinician-directed plan rather than being deployed freelance, which keeps them safe. So carry an understanding rather than a protocol, which is all this chapter was ever meant to give. You now know the shape of treatment, its several arms, and the reasoning that should govern their combination, and you know the details belong with a prescriber. That knowledge makes you a better participant in your own care, which is exactly where a book should leave you, at the threshold of a clinical relationship it has prepared you for but must not replace. With treatment understood, we can turn to the part of the journey too many people never reach, the widening of the plate, the return to a fuller life that restriction was only ever meant to serve.

Chapter 10: Widening The Plate Again

Keva got so good at the low-sulfur diet, and so frightened of losing the relief it had bought her, that she stayed on it for months past the point of any usefulness, and her diet kept shrinking, and her fear of food kept growing, and she mistook all of it for caution.

She had found real relief in a low-sulfur period, and that was the trouble, because relief that you are afraid to lose can become a cage you build for yourself. Every time she thought about reintroducing a food, the memory of how bad she had felt rose up and stopped her, and so she stayed narrow, and narrower, telling herself she was being careful. When she finally began methodical reintroduction, one food at a time with a written record, she discovered something that undid months of fear in a matter of weeks. Her tolerance had widened considerably. Many of the foods she had been terrified of caused no reaction at all. Only a couple of the highest-sulfur items still troubled her, and those only in large amounts. Her long extended restriction had not been protecting her. It had been a cage built out of a fear that reintroduction, once she attempted it, largely dissolved.

Almost every book about a restrictive diet ends at the restriction, as though narrowing the plate were the destination. This one refuses to, because the restriction was always a means to an end, and the end is a person eating a fuller, freer range of food than fear allowed them during the hard stretch.

Why reintroduction is the goal

It is worth stating plainly why widening the diet is not merely permissible but necessary, because many people, having found some relief in restriction, are frightened to loosen it and need reasons rather than reassurance.

Prolonged restriction carries real costs that mount the longer it continues. Nutritionally, a narrow diet risks shortfalls a varied one would prevent, and the low-sulfur diet in particular, by limiting proteins and a swathe of vegetables, can compromise intake if extended indefinitely (Specialists in Gastroenterology, n.d.). Beyond nutrition, a restricted diet tends to narrow the microbiome itself, reducing the diversity a resilient gut depends on, which is a quiet irony given that the whole aim was to heal the gut. And there is the human cost, the way an endless list of forbidden foods shrinks a life, complicates every meal and every social occasion, and can slide into a fearful relationship with eating that outlasts and outweighs the original symptoms. Against all of that stands the actual purpose of the restriction, which was diagnostic and calming, not curative. Having served those purposes, it has no further claim on you, and continuing it past its usefulness converts a tool into a burden. The clinician whose framing this book leans on puts it starkly, that restriction is never the endpoint and clarity is, that the goal is always to widen the diet back out and rebuild resilience (Nutrition Resolution, 2026). This gives us the principle for the chapter, and I call it the Widening Plate: the success of a low-sulfur diet is measured not by how long you can endure it but by how well you leave it.

How to reintroduce

Reintroduction done carelessly teaches you nothing and can frighten you back into restriction. Done methodically, it builds both a wider diet and a body of personal knowledge, and the whole difference is method.

The method is deliberate, one-at-a-time testing rather than a wholesale return to everything at once. You reintroduce a single food, in a modest portion, and observe your response over the following day or two before moving to the next, so that if a reaction occurs you know exactly what caused it (Nutrition

Resolution, 2026). Reintroducing five foods on the same day teaches you only that something disagreed, which is nearly useless. Reintroducing one and watching teaches you precisely which food and how much your body currently tolerates, which is the knowledge you are after. Order helps too. It is generally sensible to begin with the foods you missed most or that carry the greatest nutritional value, and to approach the highest-sulfur items, the eggs and garlic and cruciferous vegetables, more cautiously and later, since these were the likeliest triggers. A written record, as with the original trial, beats memory every time, and the appendices provide a grid for tracking each food, its portion, the day, and the reaction, so you accumulate a personal map of your current tolerance rather than a vague, shifting impression. This is exactly the map Keva built once she started, and it is what turned her fear back into freedom.

Reading reactions honestly

A hazard of reintroduction is misreading it, either seeing triggers where there are none or dismissing real ones, and since the whole exercise depends on accurate interpretation, it deserves care.

The central difficulty is that gut symptoms fluctuate for many reasons, so a bad day after a reintroduced food may reflect the food, or may reflect stress, sleep, another meal, or the ordinary noise of a sensitive gut (Nutrition Resolution, 2026). This is exactly why the one-at-a-time method and the modest portions matter, because they cut the noise and make a genuine reaction easier to spot. It is also why a single ambiguous response should not condemn a food permanently. A food that seemed to cause trouble once might be retested later, in a calmer stretch, before being written off, since tolerance is not fixed and a single bad day is weak evidence. Equally, genuine reactions should be respected rather than pushed through. If a food reliably provokes clear symptoms on repeated, careful testing, that is real information, and the right response is to set it aside for now and try again after more time and more healing, not to force it in the name of dietary freedom. The picture you build is a snapshot rather than a verdict, because tolerance tends to improve as the underlying overgrowth is addressed and the gut heals. A food that troubles you during early reintroduction may sit comfortably months later, which means reintroduction is not a one-time event but an ongoing, gradually widening process.

Handling setbacks

No reintroduction proceeds in a straight line, and setbacks are ordinary rather than catastrophic, but they are dangerous precisely because they tempt a person back into the total restriction they worked to escape, so the response to them has to be thought through in advance.

A setback during reintroduction, a stretch of returning symptoms after a food or two came back, is not evidence that the whole effort has failed or that you must retreat to the narrowest possible diet. It is information about pace, usually meaning you moved a little fast or reintroduced a higher-sulfur item before your tolerance was ready (Nutrition Resolution, 2026). The sensible response is to ease back modestly, not to the starting cage but to the level that was comfortable, let things settle, and then resume more slowly, rather than abandoning the widening project altogether. The direction of travel stays outward, toward a fuller diet, even when the pace must occasionally slow. Scotia reintroduced several foods in quick succession, hit a rough patch, and very nearly concluded she was doomed to permanent restriction. What had actually happened was only that she had moved too fast. Slowing the pace, letting things settle, and resuming one careful food at a time returned her to steady progress, and she reached a far wider diet than her frightened moment had believed possible. So hold the outward direction firmly. The plate is meant to widen. Restriction was the detour, not the destination, and reintroduction, patient and methodical and forgiving of setbacks, is how you complete the journey the diet began. With the return to fuller eating underway, we have to address the reason some people's symptoms persist despite everything, the possibility that sulfide was never traveling alone.

Chapter 11: When Sulfide Has Company

Balin did everything in this book, faithfully and well, and got most of the way better, and then stalled, and the stall nearly convinced him that everything he had done was wrong.

His sulfide-directed work had genuinely helped. His bloating eased, his gas improved, the worst of it lifted. But a stubborn residue of symptoms remained, and it would not shift no matter how carefully he stuck to what had worked, and that residue began to erode his confidence in the whole thing. If the sulfide approach was right, he reasoned, why was he not all the way better? The answer, when his clinician finally found it, was not that the sulfide work had been wrong. It was that sulfide had never been the whole story. A separate, coexisting issue accounted for the residue, one that only stood out clearly once the sulfide component had been addressed and the picture simplified. His sulfide work had not been wasted, and it had not been mistaken. It had been part of the answer rather than all of it.

Some readers will do everything here faithfully and still find themselves incompletely well, and they deserve an honest explanation rather than the implication that they must have done something wrong. Often the explanation is exactly Balin's, that hydrogen sulfide shared the gut with other overgrowths or coexisted with other conditions, and that addressing it alone was always going to leave something behind.

The overgrowths that travel together

The most common reason a well-treated sulfide problem leaves residual symptoms is that another overgrowth was present alongside it, and earlier chapters have already laid the groundwork for why.

Recall that sulfate-reducing bacteria feed on the hydrogen produced by fermenting bacteria, which links the sulfide subtype metabolically to the classic hydrogen subtype and makes their coexistence common rather than exceptional (Achufusi et al., 2020). A person may therefore have both, and addressing only the sulfide component, while genuinely helpful, can leave the hydrogen-producing partners still active. The same person may additionally have a methane component, an overgrowth of the organisms that produce methane and drive constipation. The result is a mixed picture in which treating one gas improves things partway and then stalls, exactly the frustrating pattern Balin lived. This is why experienced clinicians increasingly think in terms of the whole gas-producing ecosystem rather than a single culprit, and why comprehensive testing that examines more than one gas is so valuable when it is available (Trio-Smart, 2023). A gut is rarely running one tidy process in isolation. It is running a community, and the gases it favors reflect which members are thriving. The practical implication is not that you must chase every possible gas in a spiral of testing, but that persistent symptoms after a genuine sulfide response should prompt the question of whether company is present, rather than the conclusion that you have failed or that the sulfide diagnosis was wrong. This gives us the principle for the chapter, and I call it the Company It Keeps: sulfide overgrowth often does not travel alone, so incomplete recovery usually means unfinished business, not a wrong diagnosis.

The conditions that look alike

Beyond coexisting overgrowths, a set of adjacent conditions can mimic or accompany sulfide overgrowth, and distinguishing them matters, because pursuing the wrong one indefinitely is its own kind of trap.

Small intestinal fungal overgrowth, an overgrowth of yeast rather than bacteria, can produce overlapping symptoms and sometimes coexists with the bacterial forms, and it responds to different treatment, which is why a picture that does not fully resolve with bacterial approaches sometimes warrants a clinician's consideration of the fungal possibility (Soliman et al., 2025). Irritable bowel syndrome, under whose broad umbrella so many of these conditions have historically been gathered, overlaps heavily in its symptoms, and the relationship between the labels is genuinely tangled. Histamine-related issues, inflammatory conditions, and other gut disorders can also produce symptoms that resemble or compound the sulfide picture. I raise these not so you can diagnose yourself among them, which would be neither possible nor wise from a book, but so you understand why a clinician might look beyond sulfide when the picture is incomplete, and why that looking is good medicine rather than a sign your sulfide diagnosis was mistaken. A body is entitled to have more than one thing wrong with it at once, and the presence of a second condition does not invalidate the first. A person can genuinely have sulfide overgrowth and genuinely have something else besides, and the path to feeling well runs through addressing both, not through choosing which single label must be the true one.

Why symptoms come back

Relapse haunts this condition, and a chapter on complicated pictures would be incomplete without confronting it directly, because the return of symptoms is one of the most demoralizing experiences a person can face and one of the most misunderstood.

Earlier chapters already named the deepest reason relapse is common, that overgrowth establishes itself on a terrain of lowered defenses, and that if the terrain remains unchanged, reducing the bacterial population simply clears space for regrowth (Deloose et al., 2012). A person whose treatment addressed the bacteria but not the impaired motility that permitted them is, in a real sense, set up to relapse, not through any failure of their own but through an incompleteness in the approach. This is why the supportive arm of treatment, the attention to motility and to the underlying driver, matters so much for durability, and why abandoning it the moment symptoms ease is such a reliable route back into trouble. Other contributors include the premature abandonment of the whole plan once improvement arrives, the reintroduction of high-sulfur foods too quickly, and the reassertion of the original driver, whether a stressful period that impairs motility again or another insult to the gut's defenses. None of these is a moral failing, and framing relapse as personal failure is both inaccurate and cruel. Relapse is a feature of a condition rooted in terrain, and the response to it is to return attention to the terrain, not to conclude that recovery is impossible. A return of symptoms is a signal rather than a sentence, information that something in the fuller picture needs renewed attention rather than proof that the condition is unbeatable.

Knowing when to get help

The last question this chapter has to answer is a practical one, when a complicated or persistent picture should send you back to a clinician rather than deeper into self-directed effort, because the line between reasonable persistence and unwise solitary experimentation matters for your safety.

The self-directed work this book endorses is dietary and observational, the structured low-sulfur trial, the careful reintroduction, the honest tracking, and the assembly of a clear picture to bring to a clinician. When symptoms persist despite that work done properly, when new symptoms appear, when the picture suggests coexisting conditions, or when you find yourself contemplating the genuinely medical steps that belong to a prescriber, the responsible move is to seek professional help rather than escalate alone (Achufusi et al., 2020). And certain signs warrant prompt medical attention rather than any further self-management, and they should be stated plainly. Unintended weight loss, blood in the stool, difficulty swallowing, persistent vomiting, severe or worsening pain, or any symptom that alarms you all belong to a doctor without delay, because while they can occur in benign conditions, they can also signal something a book about sulfide overgrowth is entirely unqualified to address. No commitment to self-directed dietary work should ever override the recognition that some symptoms require a clinician now. So carry from this chapter a more complete and more forgiving understanding of why recovery is sometimes incomplete. Sulfide may have had company, in the form of other overgrowths or adjacent conditions. Symptoms may return because the terrain was never fully addressed. And a complicated picture is a reason to seek help, not a verdict of hopelessness. With these harder realities named honestly, we can turn to the wider frame that holds a durable recovery together, the connection between the gut and the nervous system.

Chapter 12: The Gut Brain Connection

Auli had addressed her overgrowth with diet and treatment, and she had improved, and then she kept sliding backward, and she could not understand why, because on paper she was doing everything right.

She had done the sulfur work. She had followed her clinician's treatment. She had reintroduced foods carefully. And still, every few weeks, the symptoms would stir again, and she would tighten her diet, and it would help a little, and then they would stir again, and the whole thing felt like bailing a boat that kept refilling. When we looked at her life rather than just her gut, two things stood out that had nothing to do with sulfur. She was living through a genuinely punishing stretch of stress, her nervous system held in a state of near-constant activation. And she grazed all day, eating small amounts every hour or two, which meant the cleaning wave that is supposed to sweep her small intestine between meals almost never got the chance to run. Adding a sustainable calming practice and spacing her meals, alongside the gut work she was already doing, steadied her in a way the gut work alone never had. Her plateau had not been a failure of the physical treatment. It had been a missing piece.

There is a temptation, in a book so focused on bacteria and sulfur and food, to treat the gut as a machine in isolation, a plumbing problem to be solved with the right inputs. That model is incomplete, and its incompleteness is one reason people like Auli plateau despite doing everything right.

The wiring between them

The gut and the brain are joined by a constant flow of signals, and understanding the rough shape of that connection makes sense of why stress and gut symptoms are so tightly bound.

The gut has its own extensive nervous system embedded in its walls, so elaborate it is sometimes called a second brain, and it is in continuous communication with the central nervous system through pathways that carry information in both directions (Deloose et al., 2012). This wiring governs a great deal of ordinary gut function, including the motility that matters so much for overgrowth. The between-meal cleaning wave, whose faltering permits bacteria to accumulate, is itself under nervous system influence, which means the state of your nervous system is not separate from your overgrowth but connected to it through a concrete, mechanical pathway. This is why the connection is more than a metaphor. When people say stress affects their gut, they are describing a real physiological relationship, not merely a mood coloring a perception. A nervous system locked in chronic activation influences gut motility, alters sensitivity so that ordinary sensations register as painful, and shapes the environment in which bacteria are either swept clear or allowed to linger. The practical upshot is that addressing the gut while ignoring the nervous system leaves part of the mechanism untouched, which is exactly what happened to Auli.

What chronic stress does

Because chronic stress is so central here, it deserves specific attention, stripped of the vagueness that usually surrounds the topic and connected to the mechanisms this book has been building.

Sustained stress affects the gut through several routes at once. It influences motility, and a nervous system held in prolonged activation can impair the very cleaning wave whose failure permits overgrowth, meaning chronic stress can be one of the drivers that lowered the gut's defenses in the first place (Deloose et al., 2012). It heightens visceral sensitivity, so a person under chronic stress may experience the same degree of gas or distension as far more painful than they otherwise would, amplifying suffering even when the underlying overgrowth is unchanged. And it shapes eating and digestion in subtler ways. This creates a difficult loop that many people with this condition recognize intimately. The gut symptoms are themselves a source of stress, worry about food, embarrassment about gas, exhaustion from poor function, and that stress feeds back into the nervous system state that worsens the gut, which generates more symptoms and more stress. The loop can spin in either direction, which is both the trap and, encouragingly, the opening, because a loop that can worsen can also be eased from either end. This gives us the principle for the chapter, and I call it the Wired Gut: the gut is wired into the nervous system through real pathways, so a durable recovery has to calm the nervous system, not only the bacteria.

I want to be careful here not to imply that stress is the cause of sulfide overgrowth or that calming the nervous system alone will resolve it, because neither is true, and overstating the mind's role is its own form of the dismissal this book has fought against. The overgrowth is real and physical and often requires physical treatment. The point is more measured, that the nervous system is one genuine contributor among several, connected through real mechanisms, and that including it in a recovery plan addresses a piece that purely gut-focused approaches miss.

Working with the nervous system

Given that the nervous system is part of the mechanism, the question becomes what can actually be done, and here the answer is refreshingly ordinary, which is both its strength and the reason it gets dismissed.

The interventions that support a calmer nervous system are not exotic. They are the unglamorous fundamentals that every source mentions and few people implement, adequate sleep, which supports both nervous system regulation and gut function, and some regular practice that shifts the nervous system out of chronic activation, whether that is a breathing practice, gentle movement, time in nature, or any approach that genuinely calms a person rather than merely occupying them. The specific method matters far less than the consistency, and the right method is the one a given person will actually sustain (Deloose et al., 2012). Meal timing connects the nervous system frame back to the gut mechanics directly, and it is worth highlighting because it is concrete and it is exactly what Auli was missing. The cleaning wave that sweeps the small intestine operates between meals, in the gaps when the gut is not busy digesting, which means constant grazing, eating every hour or two throughout the day, gives that wave little chance to run (Deloose et al., 2012). Allowing reasonable gaps between meals, without tipping into harmful restriction, gives it the space it needs to do its clearing work, and this simple structural change is one of the more directly mechanical things a person can do to support the terrain against regrowth.

The whole person

This chapter widens the frame deliberately, from bacteria and food to the whole person, because a durable recovery from this condition is finally a matter of the whole person rather than the gut alone, and saying so is not a soft platitude but a mechanical truth.

The gut is embedded in a body and a life. Its function reflects the nervous system it is wired to, the sleep the person gets, the stress they carry, the rhythm of their eating, and the general state of the organism it belongs to. A recovery plan that attends only to the bacteria and the sulfur, however well, is working on part of the system while leaving other parts, connected through real pathways, to undermine the gains, which is precisely why Auli kept sliding backward. This is why the fullest recoveries tend to come from approaches that combine the specific and the general, the targeted reduction of overgrowth and the broad support of the person, rather than from any single intervention pursued in isolation. There is also a caution to sound, one this book has raised before and returns to deliberately. In attending to food, meal timing, and the general management of a sensitive gut, a person must guard against the drift into a fearful, controlling relationship with eating and living, in which every meal becomes a source of anxiety and every choice a potential mistake. The nervous system frame can, perversely, feed that anxiety if it becomes another set of rules to enforce anxiously. The goal is the opposite, a calmer nervous system and a calmer relationship with food, and if the pursuit of gut health is generating more anxiety than it relieves, that is itself a sign the balance has tipped and that support, professional support where needed, should be sought. With the whole person in view, we arrive at the final chapter, which asks the largest practical question of all, how to actually stay well over the long term.

Chapter 13: Staying Well Long Term

Yonatan got better, genuinely and substantially better, and then spent a while feeling like a failure every time he had a bad week, until he learned to see those bad weeks for what they actually were.

His sulfide overgrowth had been calmed. His diet had widened back out to something close to normal. By any fair measure he had recovered. But a stressful stretch, or a lapse in his habits, could still stir his symptoms, and each time it happened he took it as evidence that he was not truly well, that the recovery had been a temporary reprieve rather than a real change. He was measuring himself against a standard that was never realistic, the standard of a permanent, once-and-for-all cure, and against that standard every ordinary flare looked like defeat. What finally changed his experience was not a new treatment. It was a reframe. He came to see those returns not as the failure of a cure but as the ordinary maintenance of a managed condition, and that single shift turned what had felt like repeated defeats into simply the upkeep of a life that was, by then, genuinely good.

A book like this could end at the moment of improvement, with symptoms eased and the plate widening, and leave the impression that recovery is a destination you arrive at and then inhabit permanently. That would be a comforting lie, and Yonatan's story is why I will not tell it.

What recovery actually looks like

The first task of this chapter is to correct the expectation of a clean, permanent cure, not to discourage but to prevent the disappointment that unrealistic expectations reliably produce.

For a fortunate few, treatment of sulfide overgrowth does resolve the matter thoroughly and lastingly. But for a great many people, particularly those whose overgrowth grew on a terrain of impaired motility that cannot be fully repaired, the more realistic picture is one of management rather than cure, of a condition brought to heel and kept there through ongoing attention rather than eliminated once and for all (Deloose et al., 2012). This is not defeat, and it is important not to hear it as such. Plenty of conditions are managed rather than cured, and a well-managed condition need not dominate a life. The disappointment comes not from the reality of management but from the mismatch between that reality and an expectation of permanent cure that was never realistic to begin with, which is exactly the mismatch that tormented Yonatan until he named it. Understanding this reframes the whole long-term project. The goal is not to reach a finish line and stop thinking about your gut forever, which for most people is not on offer, but to reach a state where the condition is quiet, the diet is wide, and the attention required to keep it that way is modest and sustainable rather than all-consuming. That is a genuinely good outcome, and it is achievable for many.

Knowing your own pattern

The single most valuable asset in long-term management is a deep familiarity with your own patterns, the personal knowledge accumulated across the whole journey this book has described, and it is worth consolidating that knowledge deliberately rather than letting it stay scattered.

By this point you have learned a great deal about your particular gut, which foods reliably trouble you and in what quantities, which supplements to avoid, what your early warning signs of a flare look like, what tends to precede a bad stretch, and what tools reliably help you recover. This is knowledge no clinician and no book could have given you, because it is specific to you, earned through observation and structured trial (Nutrition Resolution, 2026). Consolidating it into something you can actually consult, a personal summary of your triggers, your warning signs, and your effective responses, converts hard-won experience into a durable resource. Early warning signs deserve particular attention, because catching a flare early makes it far easier to manage than catching it late. Most people, once they look, can identify the first signals that a bad stretch is beginning, a particular kind of bloating, a return of certain gas, a dip in energy, whatever their personal early pattern is. Recognizing these early allows a modest, timely response, a brief return to lower-sulfur eating, renewed attention to meal spacing and stress, before a small wobble becomes a full relapse. This gives us the principle for the chapter, and I call it the Light Touch: once you know your own pattern, staying well becomes a light touch applied early rather than a heavy effort applied late.

A sustainable rhythm

The danger at the far end of this journey is not relapse but its opposite, the way the management of a gut condition can expand to fill a life, so that a person who is technically well spends so much energy staying well that the wellness is hollow, and guarding against this deserves as much attention as guarding against relapse.

A sustainable long-term rhythm is a light one. It involves eating a wide and varied diet, having reintroduced the foods that restriction was only ever meant to temporarily set aside, and reserving dietary caution for the specific, personal triggers that genuine testing confirmed, rather than maintaining broad restriction out of habit or fear (Nutrition Resolution, 2026). It involves the ordinary fundamentals that support the gut and nervous system, adequate sleep, some regular calming practice, reasonable meal spacing, held as sustainable habits rather than anxious rituals. And it involves responding to the occasional flare with the timely, modest tools already described, rather than treating each wobble as a crisis demanding total upheaval. What a sustainable rhythm does not involve is perfectionism, the relentless policing of every meal, the fear of every food, the sense that any lapse will trigger catastrophe. That posture is exhausting, it is usually unnecessary given how much tolerance widens with healing, and it can slide into exactly the disordered relationship with food this book has repeatedly warned against. The paradox of long-term management is that a lighter, more forgiving approach is often more sustainable, and therefore more effective, than a rigid one, because a person can actually maintain it. If you find that staying well is consuming more of your life and peace than the condition itself did, that is a signal to loosen rather than tighten, and where the anxiety around food or health has become significant, to seek support for that anxiety directly.

Living beyond the condition

This book ends where it should, not with the condition but with the life beyond it, because the whole point of everything in these pages was to return you to a fuller life rather than to enthrone a gut disorder at its center.

You began, most likely, in a place of dismissal and confusion, holding a test that said nothing was wrong while your body insisted otherwise. You have, across these chapters, gained a name for your experience, an understanding of the mechanism behind it, a way to read the test that missed it, a correctly framed dietary tool and the knowledge to use it without harm, an understanding of treatment sufficient to make you a real participant in your care, a method for widening your plate again, and an honest picture of what long-term management involves. That is a substantial transformation, from a person adrift to a person oriented, and it is worth pausing to recognize how far it reaches. But the knowledge in this book was never meant to be the destination. It was meant to be the means to a life in which the gut, quieted and managed, recedes into the background where it belongs, leaving room for everything else, for meals eaten without dread, for occasions attended without fear, for the ordinary business of living that the condition, at its worst, crowded out. The measure of your success is not how expertly you can manage your sulfide overgrowth. It is how little you have to think about it. So take what is useful here, bring the medical pieces to the professionals who should hold them, keep your personal pattern summary for the occasional flare, and otherwise let your gut do its quiet work while you get on with your life. You were never the problem, and you were never imagining it. You had a real, specific, manageable condition, and now you understand it, and understanding it was always meant to give you back the thing it had taken, which was not merely comfort but the freedom to stop thinking about your gut and start living again.

Conclusion: From Flat Line Onward

I want to return, at the end, to the person I described at the very beginning, the one holding a normal test result and feeling anything but normal, because the whole of this book has been an answer to their predicament.

The answer was not that they were imagining their symptoms, and it was never going to be. The answer was that the right thing had not been measured. There was a third gas the old test could not see, produced by organisms that consumed the very signal the test relied upon, and its overproduction accounted for a pattern of suffering that had been dismissed precisely because it fell outside the instrument. A flat line was not a clean bill of health. In the right body, alongside the right symptoms, it was the first honest evidence of what was actually wrong.

From that reframe, everything else followed. The symptoms, correctly understood, formed a recognizable pattern once the rotten-egg myth and the diarrhea myth were set aside. The tangle of sulfur words resolved into a manageable, well-defined target. The organisms behind it turned out to be ordinary bacteria that had overgrown on a terrain of lowered defenses, which meant that lasting improvement required attending to the terrain and not only to the bacteria. The low-sulfur diet, so often mishandled as a permanent sentence, took its proper place as a short and deliberate tool aimed at a wider life. The foods and supplements that backfired became specific, identifiable clues rather than a diffuse fear of eating. And treatment, testing, reintroduction, and long-term management each found their place in a coherent whole.

If this book has done its work, you are no longer the person adrift at the start. You have a name for your experience, a mechanism to explain it, and a plan to act on it, and perhaps most importantly you have the standing that comes from being believed, first by these pages and, I hope, increasingly by the clinicians you bring your clearer, better-organized picture to.

But I will end on the note this book has struck throughout, because it matters more than any fact within it. The purpose of all this understanding was never to make you an expert manager of your own gut, spending your life in vigilant supervision of your digestion. The purpose was to quiet the condition enough that you could stop thinking about it, and return to the life it had crowded out. Take what is useful here. Bring the medical pieces to the professionals who should hold them. Keep the tools for the occasional flare. And then, as far as you are able, set the whole subject down, and go and live, which is the thing this book most wanted to give back to you all along.

Appendix A: Tiered Low Sulfur Food Reference

This reference organizes common foods by their approximate sulfur content to support a structured low-sulfur trial. It is a general guide, not a personalized prescription, and your own tolerance, discovered through careful trial and reintroduction, always takes precedence over any list. Work with a registered dietitian where possible, particularly to protect adequate nutrition. Do not treat any food as permanently forbidden. The tiers describe what to lean away from and toward during a defined trial period, not a lifelong set of rules.

Higher-sulfur foods to reduce during a trial include eggs, which are especially rich in sulfur amino acids, and the allium family of garlic, onions, leeks, shallots, and chives. The cruciferous vegetables belong here as well, including broccoli, cauliflower, cabbage, kale, Brussels sprouts, and similar greens. Large portions of animal protein of any kind contribute a substantial sulfur load through their amino acids, as do certain sulfur-containing preserved and processed foods.

Moderate-sulfur foods, which many people tolerate in reasonable portions, include modest servings of various proteins and a range of vegetables that fall between the extremes. These need not be eliminated wholesale during a trial, and individual tolerance varies considerably, which is exactly why personal testing matters more than any fixed category.

Lower-sulfur foods that can form the backbone of a trial include rice and many grains, the various squashes such as zucchini, acorn, and butternut, and a range of lower-sulfur vegetables. Moderate portions of better-tolerated proteins, spread across the day rather than concentrated, allow adequate protein intake while keeping the sulfur load manageable. The aim is a diet built mainly from lower-sulfur foods for a defined period, with the higher-sulfur items eased off rather than obsessively eliminated, and always with enough total food and protein to keep the body well nourished.

Appendix B: Supplement And Additive Watch List

This list identifies supplements and compounds worth reviewing with a clinician if you have hydrogen sulfide overgrowth, because several popular supplements are significant sulfur sources that can worsen symptoms. Never stop a prescribed medication on the basis of this list without speaking to the prescriber. The purpose here is awareness, not a directive to discontinue anything on your own.

Sulfur-containing supplements most commonly implicated include N-acetylcysteine, usually labeled NAC, glutathione in its various forms, and methylsulfonylmethane, usually labeled MSM. These are frequently marketed for gut health, detoxification, and general wellness, which makes them easy to be taking without connecting them to worsening symptoms. Alpha-lipoic acid and certain other sulfur-containing compounds may also be relevant for some people.

When reviewing your regimen with a clinician, it helps to list every supplement you take, including those in combination or wellness products where sulfur-containing ingredients may be present without being obvious. Protein powders and amino acid supplements can contribute sulfur amino acids as well. The goal of the review is to identify sulfur-containing items that may be worth trialing a pause on, under guidance, to see whether symptoms improve, and then reintroducing or replacing as appropriate. As always, individual response is the real evidence, and a supplement that troubles one person may be fine for another.

Appendix C: Symptom Cluster Checklist

Use this checklist to describe your own symptom pattern accurately, not to diagnose yourself, which requires a clinician. Bringing a clear, specific account of your symptoms to an appointment is one of the most valuable things you can do, and this checklist is designed to help you assemble that account. Note which items apply to you, how often, and how severely.

Core gastrointestinal symptoms to note include bloating and its timing, abdominal pain, excess gas or flatulence, and your bowel pattern, recording honestly whether you tend toward constipation, diarrhea, or a mixture, since all three are consistent with sulfide overgrowth. Note whether any rotten-egg or sulfur smell is present in gas or burps, while remembering that its absence does not rule out the condition.

Wider symptoms worth recording include fatigue out of proportion to your rest, brain fog or difficulty concentrating, skin complaints, urinary symptoms, unusual sensations such as tingling, a general sense of feeling unwell or toxic, and heightened sensitivity to light or sound. Also record, importantly, whether you react adversely to high-sulfur foods such as eggs, garlic, and cruciferous vegetables, and to any sulfur-containing supplements, since this reactivity is a particularly telling feature.

Finally, note any test results you hold, especially a flat-line or negative breath test, and any pattern you have observed in response to dietary changes. Assembled together, these observations form a coherent picture that gives a clinician something concrete to reason about, and that picture is the single most useful thing this checklist can help you build.

Appendix D: Low Sulfur Trial And Reintroduction Trackers

These templates support the two structured experiments this book describes, the initial low-sulfur trial and the later reintroduction. Keeping a written record matters because memory is an unreliable instrument for tracking gradual change, and a written score protects you from both false hope and false discouragement.

For the low-sulfur trial, run the experiment for a defined period, commonly two to four weeks, and each day record the date, a simple rating of your main symptoms on a consistent scale such as zero to ten, and a brief note of anything relevant such as a higher-sulfur food eaten or an unusually stressful day. At the end of the period, review the pattern as a whole rather than relying on any single day, asking whether your symptoms clearly and meaningfully eased. A clear improvement points toward sulfur as a genuine driver. An ambiguous or absent response suggests looking elsewhere rather than restricting further.

For reintroduction, test one food at a time in a modest portion, and for each record the date, the specific food and amount, and your response over the following day or two before moving to the next food. Approach the highest-sulfur items, the eggs and garlic and cruciferous vegetables, more cautiously and later. Where a food seems to provoke symptoms, note it as a candidate to retest later rather than a permanent exile, since tolerance tends to widen with healing. The accumulating record becomes a personal map of your current tolerance, which is far more valuable than any generic list.

If at any point during either experiment you lose weight unintentionally, feel faint or weak, or notice restriction feeding fear or a sense of losing control around food, stop and seek professional help, because these are signs the tool has become the problem.

Appendix E: Questions For Your Clinician

Bring a concise written summary and a short list of specific questions to your appointment. A clinician who receives a clear, organized account has something concrete to reason about, whereas a rambling account invites dismissal. This appendix offers a structure for both.

For your summary, aim for a single short paragraph covering your main symptoms and their duration, any test results you hold including a flat-line or negative result, and any response you have observed to dietary changes such as reducing sulfur. Keep it factual and specific. A sentence such as a statement that you have had persistent bloating and mixed bowel habits for a stated length of time, a flat-line breath test, notable fatigue, and a clear worsening after eggs and garlic conveys more useful information than several paragraphs of apologetic narrative.

Reasonable questions to ask, framed as questions you are exploring together rather than demands, include whether hydrogen sulfide or three-gas breath testing is available or can be referred for, whether your flat-line result might be consistent with the sulfide subtype, whether a structured low-sulfur trial would be a reasonable next step to undertake together, and what could be done to support your gut motility and address any underlying driver. If you feel your concerns are not being engaged with, it is reasonable to ask about a referral to a clinician or registered dietitian with specific experience in gut overgrowth conditions.

Appendix F: Glossary

This glossary defines the key terms used in this book in plain language, for reference as you read or as you prepare to discuss your situation with a clinician.

Small intestinal bacterial overgrowth, or SIBO, is an excessive accumulation of bacteria in the small intestine, where bacterial numbers are normally kept low. Intestinal methanogen overgrowth, or IMO, is the pattern, previously called methane SIBO, in which methane-producing organisms predominate and constipation is common. Intestinal sulfide overproduction, or ISO, is the newer term for hydrogen sulfide overgrowth, reflecting that the gas is produced in both the small and large intestine.

Hydrogen sulfide is the gas, smelling of rotten eggs, produced in excess in this condition. Sulfate-reducing bacteria are the organisms that produce it, consuming hydrogen and sulfur compounds to do so, with Desulfovibrio being a frequently cited example. A breath test is the noninvasive test that measures gases in exhaled breath after drinking a sugar solution, used to assess overgrowth. A flat-line result is a breath test showing little or no rise in hydrogen or methane, which in a symptomatic person may point toward the sulfide subtype rather than confirming a healthy gut.

The migrating motor complex is the wave of muscular contractions that sweeps the small intestine clear between meals, whose impairment is a common driver of overgrowth. A prokinetic is an agent or approach that supports this motility. An empiric approach is diagnosis and treatment reasoned from the whole clinical picture rather than confirmed by a single test. Sulfur amino acids, chiefly cysteine and methionine, are the sulfur-containing building blocks of protein that contribute dietary sulfur.

References

Achufusi, T. G. O., Sharma, A., Zamora, E. A., & Manocha, D. (2020). Small intestinal bacterial overgrowth: Comprehensive review of diagnosis, prevention, and treatment methods. Cureus, 12(6), e8860. https://doi.org/10.7759/cureus.8860

Banaszak, M., Górna, I., Woźniak, D., Przysławski, J., & Drzymała-Czyż, S. (2023). Association between gut dysbiosis and the occurrence of SIBO, LIBO, SIFO and IMO. Microorganisms, 11(3), 573. https://doi.org/10.3390/microorganisms11030573

Bryan, J. (2021). Low sulphur diet: Healthy and delicious recipes on reducing SIBO symptoms. Independently published.

Deloose, E., Janssen, P., Depoortere, I., & Tack, J. (2012). The migrating motor complex: Control mechanisms and its role in health and disease. Nature Reviews Gastroenterology & Hepatology, 9(5), 271-285. https://doi.org/10.1038/nrgastro.2012.57

Lindemann, B. (2026). Hydrogen sulfide SIBO: Symptoms, testing and treatment. Bella Lindemann Functional Nutrition. https://bellalindemann.com/blog/hydrogen-sulfide-sibo

Nutrition Resolution. (2026). Low sulfur diet for SIBO: When it helps, when it doesn't, and how to use it correctly. Nutrition Resolution. https://nutritionresolution.com/

Pimentel, M., Saad, R. J., Long, M. D., & Rao, S. S. C. (2020). ACG clinical guideline: Small intestinal bacterial overgrowth. The American Journal of Gastroenterology, 115(2), 165-178. https://doi.org/10.14309/ajg.0000000000000501

Rezaie, A., Buresi, M., Lembo, A., Lin, H., McCallum, R., Rao, S., Schmulson, M., Valdovinos, M., Zakko, S., & Pimentel, M. (2017). Hydrogen and methane-based breath testing in gastrointestinal disorders: The North American Consensus. The American Journal of Gastroenterology, 112(5), 775-784. https://doi.org/10.1038/ajg.2017.46

Ruscio, M. (2024). The SIBO scenario a breath test can't detect. Dr. Ruscio Institute for Functional Health. https://drruscio.com/

Soliman, N., Kruithoff, C., San Valentin, E. M., Gamal, A., McCormick, T. S., & Ghannoum, M. (2025). Small intestinal bacterial and fungal overgrowth: Health implications and management perspectives. Nutrients, 17(8), 1365. https://doi.org/10.3390/nu17081365

Specialists in Gastroenterology. (n.d.). Low sulfur diet. Specialists in Gastroenterology. https://www.gidoctor.net/low-sulfur-diet/

Suarez, F. L., Furne, J. K., Springfield, J., & Levitt, M. D. (1998). Bismuth subsalicylate markedly decreases hydrogen sulfide release in the human colon. Gastroenterology, 114(5), 923-929. https://doi.org/10.1016/s0016-5085(98)70311-7

Trio-Smart. (2023). Unlocking ISO: Intestinal sulfide overproduction. Gemelli Biotech. https://www.triosmartbreath.com/intestinal-sulfide-overproduction

Walsh, M. (2025). Healing sulfur SIBO: The sulfur SIBO diet cookbook. Independently published.

www.ingramcontent.com/pod-product-compliance
Lightning Source LLC
LaVergne TN
LVHW022313200926
848481LV00004B/1316

* 9 7 9 8 9 0 5 9 9 3 0 7 7 *